I0448030

Lasting Weight Loss
A Quick Look

By Dr. Gary Webb

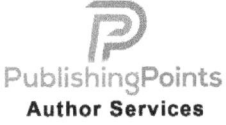

PublishingPoints
Author Services

Dalton, Georgia

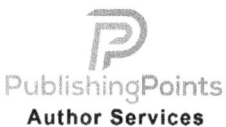

PublishingPoints
Author Services

ISBN-13: 978-1502833426

ISBN-10: 1502833425

Disclaimer

This publication is not intended to treat or diagnose any health issues. If you feel you have a condition related to this material, please contact your physician. Do not start any diet without the approval from your physician. Do not start any exercise program without the approval of your physician. If you implement any nutritional or exercise changes without consulting with your physician, you do so at your own risk. Neither the author nor the publisher assumes any responsibility whatsoever on the behalf of the purchaser or reader of these mate

Table of Contents

Introduction

This little book isn't intended to show you how to lose 100 pounds in two weeks or any of the other nonsense fads that the world is offering these days. Instead, it is intended to be a brief summary of genuine, healthy weight loss principles and practices that you can quickly implement in your own life. The results you experience will vary from one person to the next, but everyone should benefit because these new habits of eating and energizing your life have been confirmed in research studies and in the daily lives of thousands.

There is a problem built into the idea of dieting. Most of us think of a diet as two things: 1) less food for 2) a limited period of time. So we spend a few weeks, gradually getting hungrier because we think we are depriving ourselves (and we probably are); all this, just so we can fit into a new set of clothes for a special occasion. We lose the expected weight (sometimes), and then we return to the old habits of eating more and more until we weigh more than before. Those old habits die hard, especially when we don't even know which ones are defeating us. This book will seek to inform you about the habits that you need to change in order to reach and to retain your ideal weight.

Lasting Weight Loss – A Quick Look

I would love to claim some originality in the material I'm presenting, but that would certainly be dishonest. However, I can assure you that each of the ideas I've presented are ones that have been an important part of my own weight loss journey. I do acknowledge that my 60 pound loss is not sensational and may be far below what you need to lose. If you apply the principles for a longer period, you will develop those habits needed for you to reach and retain your own ideal weight.

As a word of caution, I do urge those who are reading and applying these principles to consult with their doctor about the changes in routine that they are undertaking. Your own medical condition may require some slight adjustments that your doctor will be able to recommend. My own doctorate is not in a medical field, but I've given this project my best efforts at research and have consulted with my own doctor along the way. As a Type 2 diabetic who had high blood pressure, osteoarthritis, and some knee problems, I felt that I needed his input as I was making some drastic changes in my life. Regardless of your own health circumstances, please talk to your doctor about your weight loss goals and how you are planning to reach them. If you would also like to have my personal encouragement and prayers long the way, you can contact me at gary@mgwebb.net. I am also continuing to use myfitnesspal.com. If you would like, you can join this community for free and request that I be your friend.

Chapter 1 - Goal-Setting

Goals are important for several reasons, but most importantly, you'll never know success without them. You probably already have a dream weight, one that is uniquely yours, a visual image of what you would want your body to look like. Perhaps you can imagine yourself in a bathing suit walking by your friends who are amazed to see how much better you look without all the "excess baggage" that you've been carrying around. What would that number be? How many pounds would you weigh in order to look that way? Oh, I know that other factors come into play, like whether or not you could have muscular changes to accompany the new you. But what would your dream weight actually be if you were to achieve it? Write that down right here _____. Now also write it on a card or a piece of paper to post in a prominent place, such as beside the crayon pictures on the refrigerator. Each time you see it, say it aloud, "My dream weight is..." Reinforce that dream until you begin to see it as a goal.

A dream vanishes when you wake up. A goal focuses our actions until they become ingrained habits.

My Dream Weight

My dream weight is 190 pounds. That's not what the insurance charts say I should weigh, but I don't care because I remember being that weight and didn't like it. Skinny can be just as bad as fat. I've gone so far as to search the internet until I found an ideal weight calculator that suggests that my ideal weight should be 187. Close enough! My 190 is perfect for me. I started out at 272 several years ago, but I took that down to 232 over several months. I kept it between 232-240 for about five years. Then I retired and began to gain again, back up to 250. That's when I'd had enough. My 250 looked more like 272 than 230 to me! So, I began this journey to learn all I can about weight and weight loss. I've learned a lot more than I can include in these few pages, but I'm sharing the best – just between us. Remember, my dream weight is 190, sixty pounds below the 250 level. That will ultimately also mean a loss of two pants sizes and one shirt size (actually almost two). I'm now three months into this journey, and I've hit my goal.

Six-Month Goal

A fantastic, free online source of information called *The Practical Guide: Identification, Evaluation, and Treatment of Overweight and Obese Adults* is found at this link: http://www.nhlbi.nih.gov/files/docs/guidelines/prctgd_c.pdf. If you have serious weight issues, please take time to obtain a copy and study it thoroughly.

For overweight individuals, it recommends setting a six-month goal of losing 10% of body weight. For a 250 pound man, that would be a loss of 25 pounds in six months. Since they also recommend losing 1-2 pounds per week, the 10% loss is really on the conservative side. A 2-pound per week loss over 26 weeks would be 52 pounds instead of just 25.

What do you make of all this? First, trying to lose more than 2 pounds per week can become frustrating, and even ineffective, in the long term. I've lost more in the short term, but I'm really working hard at increased activity and decreased calorie intake at the same time. Even so, I've only lost about 2.3 pounds per week on average. Be gentle with yourself when setting goals. This isn't a sprint; it's a marathon. Focus on changing your life habits to achieve modest losses on a consistent basis (about the same loss every month until you reach that dream weight).

Three-Month Goal

No, I'm not yet down to 190, but I will be if I just continue to build on the solid foundation I've already laid. And I will. By the grace of God, I will lose another 30 pounds by the end of December. Actually, that's cheating a little because at this rate, I'll probably make it by Thanksgiving.

Notice something about my three-month goal. I said I would lose another 30 pounds by the end of December. This is October 1st. I will have 13 weeks to lose 30 pounds.

5

Weekly Goals

My three-month goal of losing 30 pounds means a loss of 2.3 pounds every week! Most of the health experts say that 1.5 to 2 pounds per week is best. Some fitness trainers say that 1.5% of body weight is the maximum for athletic individuals who weigh 200 pounds or more. For me at this point, that would mean I <u>could</u> lose up to 3.3 pounds per week. My 2.3 pounds seems like a much more modest goal under those circumstances, but we should also allow for the fact that the 1.5% per week will be lower each week as I lose the pounds. By the time I'm down to 200, I will reduce my weekly goal to 2 pounds per week, spending five weeks to get rid of the final ten pounds.

Daily Goals

It would be virtually impossible to establish and succeed with a daily weight loss goal because even those who are most careful in their eating and exercising will soon discover that there are variables beyond their control. But this doesn't mean you can't have daily goals that will contribute to the ultimate, dream weight. After all, our habits are built one day at a time, with long-term repetition of the same behaviors.

I recommend that you establish at least two daily goals. First, set a goal for the maximum number of calories you plan to consume each day. If you burn the same amount of calories each day as what you eat, then you should keep the same weight. If you can burn 500 calories more, then you'll lose 1 pound per week. Got it?

I've been sedentary (a big word for lazy) until just recently. I'm a big guy at 6'3" tall. My current weight is 220 and my BMR is 2054. The BMR is the number of calories that our bodies need even if we did nothing more than lie in bed 24 hours a day.

Even my small amount of activity required 2454 calories a day (BMR X 1.2). That means I would stay the same weight if I ate 2454 calories a day. To lose 2 pounds per day, I would need to eat 1000 calories less than that or about 1454. Since I'm becoming more active over time, I'm gradually increasing the number of calories that I burn, but I'm not increasing the calorie intake very much at all. At this point, with my walking alone, I'm burning about 300 calories extra each day (raising the total to 2754). By only putting 1454 calories into my body and taking 2754 out, I'm burning up an additional 1300 calories per day or 9100 per week. Since 3500 calories burnt equals a loss of one pound, my 9100 calories will equal about 2.6 pounds per week. If I eat a few calories extra one day, it's not a disaster. I'll still hit my 2.3 pounds/week goal.

You may want to set your own weekly goal by such a formula. To do that, you can find a BMR calculator online. One of the best is found at: www.MyFitnessPal.com/tools/BMR-

<u>calculator</u>. You could also get an iPhone app called Calorie Counter Plus.

Otherwise, you can be very conservative by setting an arbitrary 1.5 to 2 pounds per week goal as recommended by many of the best fitness trainers. If you need assistance setting a sensible weekly goal, your physician is an excellent source. If you are not satisfied or don't receive the help you need, please contact me by email at <u>gary@mgwebb.net</u>.

Weighing on My Mind

Along with setting goals comes a need to evaluate progress. In weight loss, there is no escape from the need to weigh regularly – using the same scale every time. Different scales are calibrated differently so they don't give the exact same reading. For accuracy's sake, I don't even move my scale because I don't want the slightest change.

Most of the fitness gurus seem to prefer weighing at the same time on a weekly basis. They suggest that daily weighing is not advisable because it could bring discouragement to those who are vulnerable. You know your own emotional make-up better than some faceless expert, so you need to make your own choice.

I personally weigh in on a daily basis. I weigh each morning just after getting out of bed – before eating, drinking, or having any significant activity. When my weight goes down, I thank the Lord for that, but I also review the previous day's eating and exercising for clues to what might have worked. I also consider my bowel movements because that can account for some minor fluctuations on the digital scale. Some days, the scale seems to have a grudge against me. The number is higher than the previous morning. Again, I use that to review the activities of the previous day. I look at how much water I drank as well as how much I ate. I consider how much fat, protein, and carbs were a part of my total consumption. I also look at how much fiber I ate that day.

For me, the scale is an educational tool to help me spot how my habits are affecting my progress. I don't want to wait too long because I might actually forget something – even though I do record all my food, water, and exercise on the MyFitnessPal app on my iPhone.

I don't get discouraged when my weight goes up a little. I just don't want it to continue to rise for several days without me hardly even noticing.

You Need More Than a Scale

The scale isn't the only way to measure your weight loss. For some, it may not even be the most important. Another important measurement is your clothing.

Lasting Weight Loss – A Quick Look

I've had to get new pants, and I've cut my belt back a couple of inches. I started feeling a little change within a week of beginning to focus on better eating habits.

Some guys will notice a difference around the collar of a dress shirt. Ladies might see a difference in how their bra or underclothing fits.

Goals are important. As someone has said, "If you aim at nothing, you will hit it every time."

Habit-Change Goals

I want to be perfectly honest with you from the outset. Whether you lose your weight slowly or quickly is less important to me than whether you are able to reach and then retain your ideal weight. Got it?

In order for you to change your weight in a permanent way, you will need to make some permanent changes in your habits. In particular, you are going to need to find some ways to become more active, preferably ways that you will eventually find to be desirable and enjoyable. *You're looking for activities you could enjoy for the long-term, not just a few weeks.* If you hate working out with weight machines, don't do that! You are just delaying finding what will work for the long haul. Maybe you would enjoy riding a bicycle like you did as a kid. Perhaps it could be swimming, walking, jogging, playing basketball with the neighbor's kids (or better with your own). If you decide to walk, I think you might consider doing it at the mall during bad weather (just avoid stopping every time you see a "sale" sign). You might join a Pilates class or start doing some aerobic dancing. We will look into exercise in a later chapter. You might just be surprised.

You will also need to set some goals for changing how, what, where, and when you eat. Some people sabotage their weight loss by eating too narrow a selection of foods to be healthy. A strong, healthy body will burn more calories, more efficiently than a flabby, sick one. You need to begin adding foods to your regular menu (I say menu instead of diet so you don't get the wrong idea). For example, I added raw broccoli to my own food choices as a snack. I can honestly say that I wasn't too impressed with it at first, but it grows on you! I now eat it steamed as a side dish to a grilled chicken breast. Add more colored vegetables to your meal plan. You need the vitamins and minerals, as well as fiber, they supply.

You'll need to make some habit changes about how your food is prepared. Fried foods can be done well at home, using Canola spray or a little olive oil, but in restaurants, it should be classified as a hazardous waste material and carried to a disposal unit. I've had to start baking various foods and using my grill more, but I have really come to enjoy that. I also picked up one of those Nuwave® infrared convection ovens. It also has the advantage of cooking things lots quicker.

I've learned how to choose meats differently too. I could never have imagined me eating ground turkey instead of ground beef, but it's now an established routine. This change came at a fortunate time because beef has become so expensive lately. I still don't quite know how to prepare turkey burgers right, but I can make a wickedly good meatloaf, chili, and spaghetti with it. **This is how habit-change happens. One little step at a time.** There are plenty of other issues that we will consider about food changes later in the book.

Let's get started.

Chapter 2 - Why Bother?

Losing weight is not just a goal. It is a means to a better life! It's about a new future and a new you.

Are you one of the 40% of Americans who wants to lose weight? Obesity is perhaps the largest and fastest growing health threat in the nation. According to the nonprofit Trust for America's Health and the Robert Wood Johnson Foundation, 44 percent of Americans will be obese by 2030. Another 30 percent will be overweight. Is excess weight a serious matter? Is it a personal issue for you? For those who say "Yes", I hope the following pages will give you the initial jumpstart toward reaching your healthy, ideal weight.

Reasons to Lose

In weight loss, the "why" may be just as important as the "how." You may need to consider these benefits you will gain as you lose those extra pounds.

Your skin may thank you! Obesity apparently plays a role in skin blemishes and infections as well as chronic problems such as psoriasis. Studies have shown improvement in psoriasis patients who followed a low-calorie diet for just eight weeks.

You will stay more mentally sharp. According to the European Journal of Neurology, older adults who were obese performed significantly worse on tests of their mental acuity, verbal fluency, memory recall, and immediate logical memory. Apparently, excess weight makes us mentally as well as physically slower!

Your heart is less at risk. Excess weight includes several factors that contribute to additional risk for cardiovascular disease and stroke. These include impaired glucose tolerance (Type 2 diabetes), high blood pressure, and high blood lipids (bad cholesterol and triglycerides). It also seems to lead to enlargement of the left ventricle of the heart (often leading to heart failure).

You are less prone to depression. Some will argue about which comes first, the "chicken or the egg." Does depression cause people to be overweight or does being overweight cause people to be more susceptible to depression. Clearly, they often go together. Each case may be a little different. In many cases though, people who have seemed very well-adjusted and content with life have fallen into chronic, clinical depression after having gained significant weight. Some others have been able to recover from their depression by improved diet and exercise which has also led to weight reduction.

You may breathe and sleep better. According to studies from the International Society of Endocrinology, 5% of obese adults reported improved sleep after six months of weight loss. A study of 390 participants found that those who lost 5% of body weight also were able to get 22 additional minutes of actual sleep per night. That translates into more refreshed, more alert minds and bodies during the day!

You may have an improved sex life. Since your sleep quality improves with weight loss, you might just also improve in other ways between the sheets. Although Australian studies indicate improvements due to lower blood sugar in diabetics, other studies have credited improvements in heart and blood vessel functioning after weight loss. Another article, from Health.com, suggests that just having an improved self-image might account for why participants in studies report having better sexual fulfillment after weight loss. Who cares why? If weight loss makes your sex life better, isn't that what's important?

You have a lower risk for diabetes and other health-related problems. Even small reductions in weight can show improvement in blood sugar, blood pressure, cholesterol, and endocrine health. I suggest you read some of the stories on

Health.com from those who have even reversed their diabetes since making changes that produced weight loss. Greater activity plus more mindful eating habits can make a huge difference for diabetics, as well as lowering blood pressure and cholesterol.

Your cancer risk may drop. This came as a surprise to me, but both men and women have a greater risk of breast cancer when they are overweight. Women also report a greater incidence of endometrial cancer. Body fat produces estrogen, a good thing for women at some points, but too much of a good thing can bring heartache.

You are less prone to bone and joint problems. Excess weight adds pressure to joints and soft tissues of the body as well as causing inflammation that can cause great pain. USA Today reported that obese and overweight patients who have a 10% weight loss can reduce knee pain and increase walking speed. (Hellmich, 2013)

Physical activity is less difficult and more fun. If exercise and sports activities no longer hurt, you might begin to enjoy these things again. It's almost like discovering the fountain of youth. Let's face it, so much of our energy would be consumed just moving 300 pounds around that we wouldn't have much left over for jumping, spinning and all the other moves that go with an active life. Even common, enjoyable things like dancing become a burden instead of simple pleasure.

Excuses to Avoid

Now, look at some common excuses that may be holding you back from successful, lasting weight loss.

Diets make me miserable. I'm hungry all the time. I agree that a poor diet can leave you hungry. But a diet like that is poorly designed in the first place. It will not lead to permanent weight loss because you will be looking forward to going back to eating the old way as soon as it ends. A wisely planned diet will include a healthy balance of foods and reasonable portions. It will not restrict your calorie intake below 1200-1250 calories (probably not even that low). It will also include healthy snacks every two to three hours so that you aren't starving when you sit down for a meal. It will also increase the volume of water that you drink so that you don't confuse thirst with hunger. A healthy diet will cut calories, but not volume of food. In fact, you might discover that you eat more of the right things and less of those that have harmed your health for years. Another thought: Do not think of a diet as a temporary thing. Sure, you may work through some stages. I was far more restrictive in the first couple of weeks on my weight loss. Then, I made some deliberate adjustments that are still in place right now (I still have 30 pounds I want to lose). When I lose my final 30 pounds, I may make a few adjustments to help me stay there. I don't want to keep losing beyond that point. As I approach that goal, however, my rate of loss on my current eating plan should slowly decrease. I'm hoping for a smooth landing, but it may mean I add a few calories to the daily plan. I don't want to cut back on the exercise because I've come to enjoy it!

What's the use! I always just gain my weight back! Sure you do. You always will gain back the weight unless you make some permanent changes in your eating and exercise habits.   Even making small changes will make a big difference over time.   If you were to eat 300 calories less each day for a year, you would have lost 31.28 pounds. If you eat 150 calories less and burned an additional 150 calories through exercise or activity, the result would be the same.   If you were to make a permanent change of eating 500 calories less per day for the coming year, you would lose over 52 pounds. Remember, your goal isn't to see how much you can lose! It is to reach and retain your most desired weight for the rest of your life.   That permanent change of weight requires permanent changes in your habits. You can do that!

I'm too busy. Too busy to cook healthy meals. Too busy to go to the gym and work out. Too busy to plan my meals ahead. Too busy to go to a restaurant that offers a salad bar when Mickey D's is so close to work. Listen. You have time to do what you want to do most. How much time do you spend in front of the TV at night? How much time do you spend playing on the computer or messing with video games?   If you really want to change your weight, you will need to change your schedule.

I can't afford to eat healthy! The dollar menu is all you can think about when the clock is approaching 12. But you know you won't stop at $1. You'll have the fries and that over-priced soda. Maybe even a shake or an ice cream cone as you head back to work. When you total it up, that soup and salad bar might not be so expensive after all. Plus, you get what you pay for. Pay for bad health, and the fast food place will gladly deliver it at a price you think you can afford. But can you afford these days missed from work because your body doesn't have a strong immune system?

Just think of the money saved when you stop drinking sugary drinks, fat-filled chips and dips, cookies, ice cream, and pastries! Over a year's time, they represent hundreds of dollars and thousands of unnecessary calories. Nutritious fruits and unsweetened beverages can make you healthier and happier in the long run (especially after you break that sugar addiction).

Cooking at home takes too long. Cooking at home does take some time, but probably not as much as you think. The problem is that we haven't learned to plan our meals ahead and to prepare frozen meals and snacks at home. When you eat out, you can expect the restaurant to heap on the extra fats and sugars that get you hooked on a bad habit. At home, you shouldn't eat according the whims like you do when ordering off the menu. Instead, you should plan future meals while your stomach is still full from the last one. Prepare those items ahead (while you are watching TV and a timer is set). Fix several meals at a time, break them into sensible portions, and pop them into the freezer. In fact, go ahead and freeze them in microwave safe containers so that all you need to do is heat it up and eat.

I'm not the physical type; I just can't stand workouts!

You are the physical type. The problem is that your physical body is too big to move easily! If you don't start moving it now, it will just keep growing bigger. Don't buy a health club membership yet! Go for a walk instead. If you have steps at the house, go up and down those steps more often instead of stacking things up at the foot of the stairs. Do some squats and some form of a push up (even if it is just pushing yourself away from the wall. Use a gallon jug full of water or a can of vegetables as a weight to lift. Use a leather belt to help you stretch your leg muscles. The internet is full of suggestions for simple exercises. I'm planning to put together a small book of ideas myself! You may think that working out is just too hard. You are right about it being hard; that's why they call it working! You are "working out" all the fat that you've put into your system over months and years of time. It also can be hard to carry around dozens or even hundreds of extra, useless pounds of body fat every moment of every day. Those pounds of fat aren't making you stronger. They are weakening you. It's time for a change, isn't it?

My weight is because of a medical problem. Your weight may be the result of a medical problem, but it is certain to become the cause of others. If you want to be healthy, you need to lose that weight beginning today. The more you delay, the harder it will be. Talk with your doctor about what can be done to increase your calorie deficit (difference between calories consumed and calories burned). Doing something right is better than doing nothing at all. Give yourself some credit for doing all you are able to do. Don't measure yourself against the abilities of others.

If I just look at a Snickers bar, I gain five pounds! I don't know about you, but at one time not long ago that was almost true because every time I looked at a Snickers bar, I ate three of them. Don't confuse your thinking with nonsense. You don't gain weight by what you see, but by what you eat. Get the tempting items out of your house, or at least off your shelf in the frig. Someday, when you've been at your desired weight for a year, you may be able to share a Snickers with your best friend. Even then, it might be foolish to resume your old habits. Know what I mean?

21

I wouldn't have any idea where to get started. Start with what you know. You already know that some things in your refrigerator aren't healthy. Carry them to the trash! Don't give it away to some other poor soul who will begin to poison their system with it. Replace it will a variety of healthy foods and snacks. By the way, there are healthy snacks. They just aren't full of refined sugar. Try apples, carrots, celery, etc. Begin walking (if you can walk). Even someone in a wheelchair can exercise by using their arms instead of a motor to get around.

Fads to Ignore

Weight loss fads are all over the map. Most of them seem to work for at least some people in the short run, but none of them work over the long run. If you just want a temporary loss followed by a huge gain, go for it. You have a constitutional right to be stupid!

The Dukan Diet. Since it cuts out all carbs during phase 1, it will produce dramatic weight loss because it reduces sodium and causes water loss. It is a very short-term solution.

The 17 Day Diet. Same problem as the Dukan Diet.

The Atkins Diet. Same problem as the Dukan Diet.

The HCG Diet. My wife did this one. It is a ridiculous plan, including injections of HCG (human chorionic gonadotropin) and stupidly low calorie intake at 500-800 calories per day. This one could never be maintained for the long haul because it would be impossible to get a balance of nutrients from food with that small a calorie intake. The minimum suggested by almost all recognized authorities is 1200-1250 calories. I've started there and found that a very tough plan to get all my basic nutrients plus vitamins and minerals.

Cleansing Diets (such as The Master Cleanse/The Lemonade Diet, The Martha's Vineyard Diet Detox, and The Grapefruit Diet). I personally think these are the most comical. They do seem to a little sense until you look more closely. It is a quick fix with a short fuse. As soon as the cleansing stops, the weight returns. A healthy diet includes the world's original, natural cleansing agent – plenty of water. Permanent weight loss is a process of building good habits.

Ready-made Packaged Diets (like Jenny Craig, Nutrisystem, etc.) These work better than the above, but have a built in problem. They make the food choices for you, for a fee. If you want to stay on their plan for life, it would probably work for you. But it comes with the price tag of money and loss of freedom. You don't develop the new habits of choosing the better of two or three items to eat. So, when you leave the plan, you go back to your old patterns of eating because that's the power of even an old habit when you haven't replaced it with a better one.

23

Supplement-Based Diets. Forget it! Supplements can help with providing balance in your diet. I use one myself, but it isn't the basis of my weight loss. It doesn't suppress appetite or increase my metabolism. It just gives me more protein and plenty of vitamins and minerals that may be difficult to squeeze into the current calorie limits. If I cut out the supplement, I estimate that I would have to increase my daily calorie intake by about 150 calories, but I would still be losing. When I reach my desired weight, I may still continue the supplement just because of the protein helping feed my muscles after workouts.

Bottom Line:

Don't plan on fads. Don't accept excuses. Remember the great benefits that are coming for you as you continue your weight loss journey. Don't delay; start today!

Chapter 3 – New Habits for a New You
Mini-Habits

How do we establish and maintain a whole new set of habits for living, especially as it relates to lasting weight loss? It's a little intimidating, isn't it?

Let me share a secret – one that is the heart of many successes. An elephant must be eaten one bite at a time. I'm not suggesting that you add a whole elephant to your menu. I'm just saying that you can't expect to change your whole life at once. ***Doing one small thing right is better than doing nothing at all.***

Perhaps you have never done much exercise and you decide to start. Instead of enrolling at the gym and committing to spend 1 hour a day pumping iron, you could begin by deciding to do one push-up every morning for the coming year. Would that be too hard for you? You might not be able to do 100 pushups, but you could find a way to do one, couldn't you? Having done that first push-up each day, you are a success. While you are down there, you might decide to add on 10 more just for giggles! **The new habit of daily exercise begins with a small start that seems too small to fail.**

The same thing applies to your meal plans. You can't change everything in your diet all at once. **Small changes, applied repeatedly and consistently over a long period of time become habits.** That's what we're shooting for, isn't it? Let's say you want to break the habit of skipping breakfast. You might decide to begin with eating half of a whole wheat English muffin every morning before 8 o'clock. Not much of a breakfast, but it's better than nothing. Perhaps you are accustomed to drinking nothing but sweet tea at every meal. Two suggestions here: Start by mixing two containers of tea (one with sugar and the other without). Gradually start filling your glass with ¾ sweet tea and ¼ unsweetened. When you get used to that, shift to half and half; then, three-quarters unsweetened and one-quarter sweet. Eventually, you would be drinking all unsweetened tea. You might try this with some Stevia (an artificial sweetener) in the unsweetened tea. You won't taste the difference while adjusting.

If you are a sugar soft drink fan, I'd recommend shifting to the diet version of your favorite, but then plan to get off of it completely because the carbonation has some negative effects on your metabolism. If you don't care much for green vegetables, start by eating a half-portion of one at each full meal. At first you might need to add some special seasoning, vinegar, or lemon juice. You might need to stay away from some that seem a little too bitter for your taste. Do that over a long enough period, and you'll develop a taste for them. Try to eat a variety of them until you find some you like best, then occasionally go back to those you didn't care for the first time around. Our taste buds change depending on what we are accustomed to eating.

Eat for Different Reasons

Many of us have come to eat for the wrong reasons. We eat for comfort, for recreation, or for entertainment without regard for the nutritional value of what we eat. I can't deny that good food goes well with goes with good times and good friends though. Since our favorite team is playing the school rival this weekend, we stock up on the chips, dips, and sodas. We've developed the habit of associating them together in our minds. Changing the "why" we eat can have a big impact on what we eat and when. To start with, why not start with some veggies like carrots or cauliflower instead of those chips? Why not use some flavored yogurt for the dip? If you've got to have some fat, get it from some healthy nuts like almonds instead of those saturated fat chips you've grown addicted to over the years.

Let me repeat so that we don't forget it. Doing just one good thing is better than doing nothing! Repeating

one good thing for the rest of your life is better than having one success that lasts for just a season.

Value of Habits for Lasting Weight Loss

The National Weight Control Registry is the largest study ever of individuals who have lost significant amounts of weight and kept it off for over five years. The Registry does research to better understand what has produced the success of its members.

Here are some insights into how they were able to lose between 30 and 300 pounds:
- 98% of Registry participants report that they modified their food intake in some way to lose weight.
- 94% increased their physical activity, with the most frequently reported form of activity being walking.

Did you notice the one-two punch that made the difference for these weight loss successes? Both a way of eating and a new approach to activity, especially walking! Isn't that what we've been talking about in these pages?

After losing their weight, here are some of the characteristics of those who have succeeded in keeping their weight off.
- 78% eat breakfast every day.
- 75% weigh themselves at least once a week.
- 62% watch less than 10 hours of TV per week.
- 90% exercise, on average, about 1 hour per day

Again, we see a new life with new habits. Many people with weight problems neglect breakfast, but these winners don't do that. They distribute their calories evenly throughout the day, beginning early.

Those who kept the weight off were able to spot extra pounds so quickly that it just didn't get out of control.

People who kept the weight off become active participants in life instead of being spectators in front of a TV set. And look at how many devote an hour a day to exercise! I haven't gotten there yet myself. I thought I was doing well at 30 minutes. That needs to change today!

Eating an extra 100 calories a day can cause you to gain 10 pounds a year, whereas eating 100 calories less than usual may result in a loss of 10 pounds. So even a small change, for good or bad, can make a difference over enough time. That's why it is so easy to slide backward after being successful in losing weight. Let's develop the habits that lead us in the right direction. Okay?

I want to learn from the people who know how to succeed at making their dream weight into a reality and keeping it that way. Don't you?

Physical Fitness: Making Exercise a Habit

Making exercise a habit for those of us who have been sedentary for a long time is not an overnight event. It is a slow process. Actually, I messed up some and slowed my own progress by jumping into exercise with both feet, literally. Even though I had become a couch potato, I started trying to run a mile each day and work out for 30 minutes on exercise machines at the gym. Guess what? I messed up one knee that just couldn't handle it. The body has its ways of just saying "No!"

The habit of daily exercise is vital for lasting weight loss. If exercise is ever going to become a habit for you, you'll need to start thinking about it just like brushing your teeth or taking a daily shower. It should be automatically included because you realize you need it in order to live a better and more enjoyable life.

I now would say that we need to set realistic goals and take small steps to fit more movement into our daily lives. For example, we can begin by fitting short bursts of activity into our schedule, things like taking the stairs instead of the elevator. We can do a short series of exercises, like leg lifts (bringing our knees as high up and as close to our chests as possible). Many other "body weight" exercises are available through the Net. See Appendix B.

To **add variety to your routine**, which will help you stay with it. Why not change up the daily routine by swimming one day and doing some power walking the next? Or, work out your legs one day; and your upper body the next.

Bottom Line:

I'm glad you are reading this book, but don't spend all day doing that when you need to put it into practice piece by piece as you learn. Get up and go do one good thing instead of nothing!

Chapter 4 - Wash Away the Pounds

Let me ask you a question. I'm sure you know the answer though. "How many calories does water have?" None. Let me ask another question that you can answer, but I can't. "When was the last time that you drank at least a full 8-ounce glass of water?" Was it more than two hours ago? Danger! You are dying of thirst!

Your Body is Thirsty

When you are trying to lose weight, the most important ingredient in weight loss is water. Why? Because **the first weight you will be losing is mostly water.** You are likely to feel so proud of yourself that you have lost five pounds in just four days, but you are actually hurting yourself in the long run. You are becoming dehydrated, so your body is not working as well as it should. You cannot burn calories efficiently without plenty of water. In fact, dehydration slows down your metabolism.

Cleansing, The Healthy Way

Burning calories is like burning gasoline or diesel in a vehicle. We've all heard about the pollution coming out the exhaust, haven't we? What if the carbon dioxide and other pollutants couldn't escape from the engine? It would soon cease to work because it could no longer process its fuel. Burning calories produces toxins that must be eliminated from your body or the body will begin to die. Some will be eliminated by perspiration, some by respiration, some by urination, and some by defecation – all of them requiring water to carry some of the polluting toxins from your system.

Water is essential for proper functioning of the fiber in your food. Without enough water, that fiber that would normally contribute to bowel regularity actually cause constipation (not good for your weight).

Medicine for Your Muscles

Then, there's your muscles to consider. Without enough water, you won't have enough blood to carry oxygen to your muscles. Without the oxygen, your muscles will accumulate gases that make you feel more tired (unlikely to exercise much, huh?). Water also lubricates your muscles and connecting

34

tissues, as well as your joints so that you will become less sore after that workout.

Fullness Minus Fat

Drinking 16-ounces of water thirty minutes before a meal will fill you up and cut your calorie consumption significantly. Drinking it during your meal will cause you to feel full much sooner.

How Much Is Enough?

Many fitness gurus recommend drinking eight 8-ounce glasses of water every day. I personally drink over 120 ounces per day (but I started off at 252 pounds). To lose weight, don't drink less than the recommended amount. Consider, however, that some of your drinks contain water, but also cause you to expel water because they contain caffeine. Coffee, tea, and most soft drinks contain lots of caffeine (especially Mountain Dew and the so-called energy drinks).

The Mayo Clinic recommends a formula to calculate how much to drink. If you are not very active, you should multiply your weight by one-half to determine how many ounces to drink. That's the way I did because I was so sedentary. If you are more active (which I soon became after beginning to lose weight) then you should divide by two-thirds. That would mean I should be drinking about 140 ounces per day, especially when I'm going to be doing a lot of aerobic activity like running.

Sometimes, when we feel hungry, we are actually thirsty. That's because we assume that nerve signals coming from our stomach must mean we're hungry. **Start drinking a glass of water when you seem hungry within two hours of having eaten a meal or a snack.**

If the temperature and humidity is high, and you are being more active than usual, you should increase your water intake. If you are perspiring heavily, then you need to drink Gatorade, Powerade, or something similar to replace electrolytes.

If you feel thirsty, you are already dehydrated. Try to spread out your water consumption throughout the day. I've even noticed that on the few days when I didn't get enough of my water because I waited too late in the day, I also gained weight. I'm not sure this applies to everyone, but it only makes sense to drink throughout the day to stay hydrated. Other than thirst, you have another indicator of dehydration: urine color. If your urine is pale yellow or clear, then you aren't dehydrated. A darker color could also come from some vegetables like asparagus.

Many advertisements offer a beverage to start your day. **For weight loss purposes, nothing beats starting the day with 16 ounces of water!**

Bottom Line:

Start keeping track of how much water you are drinking each day. Maybe use your smartphone as a convenient place to record each 8 ounce serving. Avoid sugar based drinks like colas or other drinks that have high fructose corn syrup.

Chapter 5 - Eat More Food, More Often

It may surprise you, but you might not be eating enough to have lasting weight loss. You can actually eat so little that your body will move into "starvation mode" and begin to conserve a high percentage of your calories by storing them as fat.

Some people are not eating enough of the foods our bodies need. Over time, those with weight problems tend to eat a narrower selection of foods, but in larger and larger quantities. The food they are eating just doesn't do the job when it comes to satisfaction and health. Our appetites are governed by physical things like hormones and by psychological things like using food to meet emotional needs.

Maybe You're Hungry Because of Hormones

Ghrelin – the hunger hormone. This originates in the gastrointestinal tract and signals the hypothalamus and brain that we are hungry. Ghrelin levels rise immediately before time to eat, but they drop quickly after we eat. Even a small amount of food can cause ghrelin levels to start falling. Important! You don't have to keep on eating. Eat a little and then stop. Give your body a chance to catch up and to reduce the ghrelin levels.

Leptin – the fullness hormone. Leptin is produced by fat cells and regulates the amount of fat stored in the body. In morbidly obese patients, this hormone can be very high, but still not reduce the person's hunger. Weird. That means that we can so cripple our systems until the normal process of hunger relief by eating does function properly any more This condition of "leptin resistance" means we can still be hungry on a full stomach.

Hungry People Tend to Eat More Than They Need

Food meets the needs of our bodies for health and energy. But that doesn't stop us from trying to use food to meet other needs. If we are bored or lonely, the refrigerator can become our friend. We can use food to soothe our pain during stressful times. We can eat mindlessly while watching TV or playing games.

Don't allow yourself to be hungry.

Before the ghrelin (hunger hormone) begins to drive your cravings, go ahead and eat something. That will help shut it down before your appetite begins to rage. I've learned that **it is important to eat regularly throughout the day**. This distributes the calories and gives the body a maximum benefit from the nutrients needed. As a diabetic, it helps keep my blood sugar even. In fact, as I'm losing weight, the blood sugar has become less of an issue at all. I eat five times a day: three meals and two snacks. Small nutritious snacks accompanied by a glass of water will help to curb our cravings and help us avoid overeating. **Make it a habit to eat often throughout the day, just learn to choose some low calorie snacks.** More about that later.

Understand the Major Nutrients in Your Food

To have better eating habits, you need to understand how food works in your body. Not technical details about various amino acids that produce protein. Not about the omega-3, 6, 7, or 9 acids in fat-laden foods. Not about the mono- or polysaccharides that form simple carbohydrates. But you need to know the basics in order to be able to read labels on various foods and make better choices for this day forward. **You only need to understand enough so that you can consistently make wise food choices.**

<u>**Proteins**</u> **are crucial in the body for building, maintaining and repairing body tissue, especially muscle and our vital organs**. Since muscle tissue constantly needs repair, we must have a regular supply of protein to maintain our physical strength. In addition, all enzymes and hormones are proteins that maintain the health an vitality of our bodies.

Furthermore, proteins aid in our resistance to various disease bacteria and viruses.

Fat **provides protection for the body.** Fat insulates and maintains body temperature and cushions to protect body organs. It also promotes growth and development, as well as maintaining cell membranes, including the nervous system and brain. Fat also plays a crucial role in the digestion of fat-soluble vitamins such as vitamins A, D, E, and K. All these need fat in order to be absorbed into the body.

Carbohydrates **are our main energy source.** They consist of chains of small, simple sugars that are broken down and enter the body as glucose. One sugar, called glucose, is essential for the body, as it is the preferred source of energy in our brain, heart and central nervous system. A more complex carbohydrate is starch. The starch must be broken down in the intestines into sugars that the body can use directly. One form of carbohydrate, called fiber, is not digested into the body. **Fiber aids our intestines in expelling waste and can help lower blood cholesterol.**

You need a good balance of all these foods in order to maintain long-term health. Many fad diets treat either fats or carbohydrates as if they are evil, but both are needed. I am personally using a 40-30-20 percentage of carbs, protein, and fats. However, the experts still don't seem to agree about what are the best levels.

The Habit of Healthy Food Choices

Healthy food choices cannot be made without solid information about the portion size, calorie level, and major nutrients in the food being considered.

Portion Size. Those with chronic weight problems do not have the habit of measuring or weighing the foods they eat. Nor do they have a good way to estimate portions when eating away from home. Packaged goods at home normally give you the number of servings included in the can or box. While at home, it is wise to use a good measuring cup to select your portions. On some occasions, a kitchen scale would also be helpful.

Here's a little chart to help you estimate portions of food

Measuring Size.....................Equivalent

Measuring Size	Equivalent
1 Cup	A baseball
½ Cup	A light bulb
¼ Cup	A large egg
1 Tbsp	End of Thumb
1 Tsp	End of Index Finger
3 Ounces	A deck of cards

These are some of the common sizes of food portions recommended in recipes and on food labels.

43

Calorie Level. Some foods are calorie dense. By that, I mean that a small quantity of the food can yield a high number of calories. You should develop the habit of choosing foods that offer a smaller amount of calories for the portion size and the nutrient mix. After you reach your ideal weight, it will be even more important for you to learn about what portion sizes of various foods you can eat without adding too many calories or too many fats.

Grams of Major Nutrients. As you read a label or use an app like MyFitnessPal, you will notice that the quantities of fat, carbohydrates and protein are listed in grams. But just remember that one gram of fat produces three times as many calories as a gram of carbohydrates or protein. So, don't try to have equal amounts of each or you will have food that is full of fats. Also notice that the fiber is included in the number of carbohydrate grams, but it does not produce any calories because it isn't digested.

Learn to eat healthy snacks

Snacks once meant something different for me. A king-sized Snickers bar and a large Diet Coke were almost a reflex. Now, it's low-sodium turkey jerky, a hard-boiled egg, a deli roll-up, or another snack from the cabinet. Strange things can happen, though. I'm not suffering. I can eat a frozen protein Creamsicle or a frozen yogurt for just a few healthy calories. I can enjoy a big bowl of air-popped popcorn sprayed with aerosol butter flavored oil. I really love the low-fat cheese sticks that are only 50 calories. The homemade dried apples I was given by a friend turned out to be wonderful!

Some of the fad diets warn against fruits like oranges or bananas because they are filled with natural sugars. Sorry 'bout that! They taste good; they are filled with nutrients I need and the number of calories isn't that high after all. Apples even make a great breakfast food when I slice them up, sprinkle them with cinnamon, and stick them into the microwave for a couple of minutes. I haven't tried that for a snack yet, but I'm sure I'll get around to it. Those little gelatin cups sold at Walmart are a fantastic treat for just five calories. Or, maybe I should just settle for a frozen Jello Pudding Pop. It's only 60 calories, and I do love chocolate.

Just a little warning though. I love raisins and dried cranberries, but they are calorie-packed. A cup filled with raisins has eight times the number of calories as the same sized cup filled with grapes. Just be careful with your portions on things like that!

Be sure to check out Appendix C for a list of low calorie snacks.

Bottom Line:

You don't need to starve yourself to lose weight, but you do need to know what foods and what quantities are best for you to build into your meal plans.

Chapter 6 - Eat Differently

It seems obvious that we can't keep on eating like we've been eating but expect different results. We've gained weight because we have a habit of eating the wrong foods in the wrong quantities, at the wrong times.

Eat a Greater Variety

Since I've been studying weight loss, I've noticed something that hasn't been mentioned directly by any of the books or speakers. The people who are overweight don't eat as big a variety of foods as those who are slender. As we become addicted to sugars and fats, we eliminate the foods that don't have an abundance of it. Our taste buds become tuned to that sugary taste, that salty taste, that greasy flavor, instead of delighting in healthy, natural flavors.

Many of us who are overweight have a tendency to eat too few of the colored vegetables like greens, asparagus, broccoli, carrots, squash, etc. We eat less fish and chicken when compared with beef and pork. We eat more fried foods and less baked or grilled. We need to make a change here!

47

It was only a few months back that I discovered the common denominator between some of the foods I didn't like. Things like cilantro in salsa ruined it for me. Why? Because cilantro is a bitter herb. I don't naturally like anything with a bitter edge to it. Not chicory or basil. Not endive or turmeric. Certainly not dark chocolate, some dark coffees, or chamomile.

But bitter foods have benefits as well, so I know that I need to eat more. They help the body to absorb nutrients by stimulating gastric juices in the stomach. Eating at least some of the mild bitter foods can help us to avoid having "sweet tooth" cravings. They help the body to detoxify, especially the liver.

I've actually learned to enjoy one bitter flavor – green tea. Now, I find out that green tea helps to stimulate our metabolism by as much as 4%. Green tea also inhibits fat absorption, so it is good to drink it when you have eaten something with too much fat.

Eat More Raw and Unprocessed Foods

Do most, if not all, of your grocery shopping around the outer edges of the grocery store. Why? Because that's where they locate the refrigerated foods and the natural, unprocessed foods. That's where you'll find the fresh vegetables, meats, fish, eggs, and milk. These are foods that come to you from nature, without a processing plant in between. The boxed and canned stuff is in the aisles instead. Most of these processed foods contain added salts, sugars, and fats as well as chemicals to preserve them. Unprocessed foods will get their processing as you prepare them and eat them. Your body knows what to do with real food. The phony, processed foods are often difficult for your body to process properly. In addition, some of them are just concentrated calories that your body can send directly to your fat cells.

Unprocessed and even raw vegetables have more of the nutrients intact, so your body's needs become satisfied with less food. Some hunger comes from bad nutrition. We've eaten a large quantity, but that heavy plate didn't hold the basic nutrients that our body needs to function well, protect itself against disease, and to convert food into energy.

Eat Well, without Trying

Stop eating from boxes and bags. If it isn't worth putting on a plate or in a bowl, don't eat it. I know we're all into convenience, but when you eat from the container you got from the store, there's no thinking involved in the quantity that you eat.

Control your portions by using smaller plates. Dinner plates have gotten larger and larger since I was a child. I recommend that you begin eating from smaller plates and bowls, so that your portion control is built in.

Stop eating refills. One well-loaded plate should be enough. One piece of meat is enough. One trip to the salad bar should be enough. While you are still trying to lose weight, one trip to the dessert bar is too much!

You Get What You Pay For

I mentioned earlier that people often complain that eating healthy is too expensive. In a way, they are right. The foods are more expensive by volume, but you'll be eating less volume when you eat healthier. You'll be able to get the nourishment your body needs instead of the stuff your body has been conditioned to crave. You also need to understand that you may be paying for the inexpensive food in other ways, including bad health.

As a child, we didn't have much, but my mom was a mistress of stretching a nickel into a dollar. I didn't develop an exotic taste in foods because that stuff wasn't on our menu. As an adult, when it came to food choices, I tended toward getting whatever was cheapest – either at the grocery stores or in restaurants. Now, I realize that many of those least expensive foods are very expensive when it comes to the damage to our bodies. I would have always picked an inexpensive buffet over a "good" restaurant at the same price. Why? Most food for the money! As if I was in need of more food! What I've needed was better foods prepared in better ways.

Bottom Line:

If you keep on eating like you've always been eating, then you will keep on getting the results you've always gotten. If that's what you want, go for it! But remember that a temporary change in your eating will only bring a temporary change in your weight.

Chapter 7 - Get a Move On

If I had it my way, exercise wouldn't be necessary to maintain a healthy body. You can call me lazy, but I just don't like the idea of spending lots of time doing things I don't like doing and getting nothing from it.

When I was a teen, I was skinny. We lived out in the country, so I didn't exercise. I worked. I put up hay and tobacco for one of our neighbors. I cut, hauled, and stacked hundreds of loads of firewood during the long East Tennessee winters. I didn't play football or basketball because I had too many chores to do at home before sunset. Needless to say, I was deprived of the opportunity to exercise. But I was six foot three inches tall and weighed 160 pounds. I was just skinny legs and bony brown arms. In fact, the small town nearest to our home didn't even have a fitness center. For that matter, I'm not too sure the larger towns did either. People were just too busy to exercise in those days, and they sure wouldn't have wanted to pay to do it. You see **exercise is a lot like work except you don't get paid to do it.**

Or do you? Exercise does pay, especially for those who don't get up early and work late at very physical jobs. That's most Americans these days. We think we are pretty smart because we get paid to think instead of building callouses on our hands and coming home with sore backs. We probably are smarter in some ways, but we don't really know how to keep our bodies from ballooning with the fat we've accumulated by sitting behind a desk all day. Our bodies have become weaker and weaker, so how smart are we?

Enough of the sarcasm. Let's get to work. **If you are like the 44% of Americans who are already overweight or obese, then you don't burn as many calories each day as you put into your body!** Perhaps you've tried all the fancy fad diets, but eventually you discover that something's just not working. **Even if you've begun to develop better eating habits, you aren't making the progress you expected in weight loss.** Perhaps you also realize that you won't be able to spend the rest of your life just eating celery and carrots. You'd like to add a steak to your plate once in a while instead of always eating chicken, fish, or no meat at all. Reality is: **There is no lasting weight loss for couch potatoes.**

If you want lasting weight loss and a well-balanced menu, then you will have to get a move on. **You are going to have to start doing some things that burn calories faster than you are putting them in your mouth.** I don't mean that you will have to join the local fitness club and pay a year's dues. You just need to get up out of that recliner, turn the TV off, and do something that pushes your body and its metabolism into high

54

gear for a few minutes to an hour every day. I repeat. **If you are going to experience lasting weight loss, a change of eating habits is important, but not enough. You must get into the habit of doing some energy-burning exercise on a regular basis for the rest of your life. Exercise is probably less important than food consumption for weight loss, but it is at least as important as your eating habits for long term weight control.**

I remember a friend who used to say, "I'll just have a small piece of pecan pie, and then I'll go exercise it off later." Then, she'd take a slice that was a fourth of the whole pie, probably a thousand calories. Later she might take a ten minute walk, thinking that would take care of the 1000 or so calories in the pie. She must have not been very good with math. At 150 pounds, her ten minute walk burned 34 of that 1000 calories. And she didn't understand why her pants were getting larger every year! **Again, you cannot have lasting weight loss just by restricting what you eat, nor can you just do a minor amount of exercise to make up for poor eating habits. It must be both sensible eating <u>and</u> consistent exercise.**

Get Moving with Cardio Exercise

The American Heart Association recommends that everyone should get at least 20 minutes of <u>vigorous</u> cardio exercise (like jogging or running) three times a week, or at least

30 minutes of more moderate cardio (like walking or mild bicycling). If you have health issues like high blood pressure, heart disease, or stroke history, you should definitely check with your doctor before increasing your activity beyond your normal levels. You should also plan to spend 5-10 minutes before and after exercise just warming up or cooling down.

Calculating Your Target Heart Rate for Cardio

For cardio (aerobic) exercise, you should plan to get your heart pumping above its normal range. To estimate your target heart rate, here's a simple formula: Subtract your age from 220, then multiply by 0.7. As an example for a 50-year-old man the calculation would be (220-50)=170, 170x0.7=119. So, 119 would the target heart rate for such a man. Let me add one condition. If you are using some medications (particularly for heart related problems), consult with your doctor because he might want to make some adjustments to accommodate your changing exercise level.

Cardio vs. Strength Exercises

Many people think that weight control only benefits from cardio exercises. Obviously, cardio does burn more calories during a single session, but that's not the full picture. Strength exercise builds muscle. Muscle does two things for your goal. It will make you appear more slender even when you weigh a little more. Secondly, since muscle burns more calories than fat cells, you will actually use up more calories throughout the day if you build more muscle.

Cardio exercises include longer periods of running, bicycling, hiking, skiing, and swimming. Strength exercises include shorter periods of weightlifting, calisthenics, Pilates, or body-weight exercises like pull-ups. Cardio should be considered as a daily activity with some variety in what is being done. Try to make it something you really enjoy doing. Strength training should be 2-4 times per week with some recovery days between periods of hard workouts.

A Simple Plan for Cardio

With cardio, you should try to extend yourself more and more over time. **Begin with fast walking.** I know that some of us are confirmed couch potatoes. Walking is a good start and can be moved forward by walking faster and farther over time. In fact, you could also add a heavy backpack and head toward the mountains!

Try interval training. Interval training will allow a great calorie burn and will help extend your workout time, regardless of the activity you are pursuing. Here's how. Push yourself really hard for one minute, then ease up some for a couple of minutes.

Extend your workout time. As a beginner, 20 minutes might seem like a lot, but you should seek to gradually increase your ability to 45-60 minutes per session over time. When you do this, those extra minutes will actually be more effective in burning fat than the early part of the workout.

Heat it up. Begin to increase the difficulty of what you are doing. Run harder; tilt the treadmill incline more, increase the weight on the gym equipment, etc. Push outside your comfort zone at least a little. That extra effort will release endorphins (chemicals in the body that relieve stress and ease pain).

Strength Training at the Gym or Living Room

Muscles don't become stronger until they need to do so. Only after muscle fibers begin to stretch and tear do they start to grow thicker and stronger. That doesn't happen with our regular routine. We need to add some weight to our activity. It can be something as simple as using a full gallon jug like a kettle bell, using a can of beans for working your triceps with a "kickback" exercise, or using a broom handle to work out your forearms. Stairs can be used to tone and strengthen those calf muscles. This book doesn't focus on this single aspect of the subject, but a future one probably will be. Weight training doesn't require a gym membership or a roomful of expensive equipment. If you would like to know more about simple body-weight exercises or other inexpensive approaches, you can find 25 great exercises on the web at http://www.acefitness.org/acefit/fitness-programs-article/2863/Top-25-At-Home-Exercises/.

However, I will credit many fitness clubs with providing the motivation and resources needed for beginners to see rapid muscle growth. I'm fortunate enough to have found one that is operated by a local Presbyterian church. It only costs $75 per year. Similar programs exist in many cities.

Get Moving, but Don't Get Bored

If you get into a rut by doing the same old routine every day, you may lose interest and quit. It's just a human problem of motivation. You've got to keep a little spice in the process. Try new things from time to time. In fact, some things that you hate the first time you try them may become favorites after the third or fourth attempt. When you get well toned, you might even jump into something like Zumba or other fast paced dance program. Or you could shift to a sport like racquetball, tennis, or one-on-one basketball or volleyball. The only limit is our imagination and motivation. Let's get moving here!

Don't be a Lone Ranger

I'll say more about this later, but let me go ahead and say that some people make little progress with becoming more active without enrolling in some kind of exercise class or even getting a personal trainer for a few sessions. In most cases, a few classes are enough. Personal trainers are often too expensive, so I've never had one.

A Final Word

Don't exercise while dehydrated. It will weaken your workout intensity and also make your fatigue increase rapidly. Dehydration also interferes with metabolism, so you will lose much of the benefit you were expecting from your workout. In fact, I recommend consuming about 16 ounces of water about 15-30 minutes before starting the workout. Then, also drink a few sips frequently as you exercise.

Bottom Line:

You might lose some weight with very little exercise, but you are very unlikely to keep it off without adding more challenging activities to your life.

Chapter 8 – Dealing with People
Just a Little Help from My Friends

Let me begin with an obvious statement. Change often produces conflict and stress in relationships. Both eating and physical activity have a social impact. Those who are closest to you may be the ones who most oppose the changes you are trying to make in your schedule, eating habits, and daily activities. They could also be your most helpful supporters. It is best to get them on board early in your new efforts to reach and retain lasting weight loss. Some may be willing to endure a short period of changed eating, but not a lifetime. They want things to go back to "normal".

For some families, eating together is the only significant time of interaction. That isn't healthy, but we are talking about reality instead of the ideal. If you have children, I would encourage you to get active in ways that include them. It could be something as simple as tossing a ball around in the back yard or as ambitious as a ten-mile backpacking trip in the mountains. If your kids or your spouse are slower than you, be very patient, but keep yourself active. Build physical activity into your relationship, or else it will eventually disappear.

Perhaps you and your spouse could join a fitness club together, even if she's doing Pilates while you are doing a cardio bike. As time passes and you both grow stronger, the possibilities for having fun together will increase. You might start riding bicycles together, taking long walks in the park together, or canoeing on the weekends. Gradually, you can become a participant in life rather than a spectator.

Beyond your family and closest friends, you can begin making new friends on your weight loss journey. As an example, you could join a number of different classes in a fitness club. You and your spouse could join a dance class to work off some calories and also get ready for a vacation.

At first, you might also want to join a group like Overeaters Anonymous or Weight Watchers. There, you find the support of others who are familiar with the struggles you are going through. Some churches also sponsor programs for those battling lifelong weight problems. Local hospitals in some cities have developed community outreach programs focused on weight control. Any of these can connect you with someone who understands and is able to offer support.

You can even find new friends online. There are many only support groups for those trying to lose weight. Many of them include people who have already lost 100 pounds or more.

Bottom Line:

The battle is yours to win, but you don't need to fight it all alone. Friends and family may or may not be supportive, but it's best to help them understand the long-term nature of your efforts. They need to understand that you are building new habits, not just trying something for a little while.

Chapter 9 – Sliding to a Finish
The Glide Path & Overkill Principles

There is no victory lap for weight loss. It is a lifetime process. I have seen many people decide to "reward" themselves after reaching their ideal weight. How? By going out to their favorite restaurant and indulging themselves in all the foods they've missed during the period of weight loss. That is utterly ridiculous! If you really believe you've been eating wisely, why change? Why eat foolishly as a reward? Bad eating should be considered a way to punish your body, not a reward!

The Glide Path

During the final weeks as you approach your ideal weight, you should become especially observant about what and how much you are eating. I've already said that you should be recording everything that goes into your mouth, but during this period it becomes even more significant. During the time of weight loss, your body has adjusted to the changes you've been making. It is doing more with less. That means that a sudden increase in calorie input will be stored because it just isn't needed. In those final weeks, you need to re-calculate your BMR based on diminished weight and higher level of activity. It may well be that you can increase your calorie input, but you will still need to set a reasonable limit.

The same applies to exercise. You will need to solidly establish your exercise habit or it will slip away once you reach that magic weight number. Get a friend to hold you accountable and to join you in your workout plan. Don't slow down.

Overkill

My recommendation for everyone is to establish a buffer by going below your weight goal by 5-10 pounds. You may well need that margin while you are seeking to find the best calorie level and nutritional mix to maintain your goal. Consider the three month period after reaching your goal as the "red zone." You haven't really made a touchdown yet, but you are close. Carefully evaluate your eating and exercise habits <u>after</u> you hit the ideal weight you set at the beginning of this book. You could even use something like Appendix A as a checklist of habits that you might want to make permanent.

You Win

After you've kept the weight off for a few years, you should understand the habits you've learned and applied much better. You'll have your own customized health and fitness plan. You have won the game... or have you? Let's go check the scale one more time. Maybe you should pull out the tape measure to check your weight.

Bottom Line:

If you ever need to get a bigger pair of pants or a longer belt, you should accept the truth and start back at

the beginning. Old habits die hard, and new ones can quickly fade away.

Appendix A
Quick Summary of Habits for Weight Control

Do these simple things in order to lose weight. Most of them will need to be continued if you want to keep it off.

1. **Always remember the Five Word Diet Plan:** It's simple. *Eat less, but Move More!*

2. **Start drinking more water.** Gradually add more each day until you reach one gallon per day. Ice water also has the advantage of increasing metabolism (the rate your body burns calories). Drink 8-16 ounces before each meal. Drink at least 8 ounces during the meal. Don't wait until you are thirsty to drink; that's too late.

3. **Calculate your Basal Metabolic Rate.** Either use an online calculator or the (less accurate) formula here. Women: BMR = 10 times current body weight. Men: BMR = 12 times body weight.

4. **To lose one pound per week, deduct 500 calories per day from your BMR.** To lose two pounds per week, deduct 1000 calories per day from your BMR. This is your maximum amount of calories per day to lose weight at the desired rate. Do not set a calorie limit below 1250 per day.

5. **Start reading labels and limiting calories to reach your daily goal.** Remember one gram of fat produces three times more calories than one gram of protein or carbs.

6. **If you can't pronounce the ingredients, then don't eat the food.** When you look at the label, read the ingredients carefully. Most chemicals have long, complex names that are a little scary... for good reason. Be very afraid! Stay away!

7. **Only shop with a full stomach.** If not, those fats and sugars will look irresistible. Shop from a list that you have prepared before arriving at the grocery store.

8. **Record what you eat and the amount.** Do this in a paper diary or with an app like MyFitnessPal. It's available at the App Store, Google Play, or on the internet at www.myfitnesspal.com.

9. **Record your progress.** You could do that with a little poster in the bathroom (right by the scale). Or you could add those progress entries into MyFitnessPal. I'll admit it; I love that app!

10. **Eat on a schedule, instead of feeding your cravings.** Eat something (even just a little) every two to three hours. Never allow yourself to get really hungry. Between meal snacks (mid-morning and mid afternoon) help prevent overeating at mealtime. Keep

your shelves and refrigerator stocked with nutritious, low fat, low calorie snacks.

11. **Count your calories before you eat them, not afterwards.** In my case, I sometimes consider eating something, plug it into MyFitnessPal, and then change my mind when I discover that it has more calories than I thought. Bottom line: Plan your meals before meal time.

12. **Never skip breakfast.** That will kick start your metabolism and also help ensure that your calories are better distributed throughout your day. Eighty percent of those who have been able to maintain a weight loss of at least 30 pounds for at least a year report that they always eat breakfast. (Johnson, 2012)

13. **Eliminate fatty fried foods and high sugar foods.** Increase use of protein-rich and complex carbohydrate foods. If you see high fructose corn syrup, high up on the list of label ingredients, RUN!

14. **Add more fiber to your meals,** even if that means using a fiber supplement, and drink plenty of water with it so that it helps bowel regularity.

15. **Eat from individual plates or bowls while sitting at a table.** Leave the serving bowls in the kitchen, and don't go back for seconds. Make sure you are eating from a 9" plate instead of a large one.

16. **Store all food in the kitchen and pantry.** Make these areas off limits after your evening meal.

17. **Understand "diet foods."** Most of them compensate by replacing sugar with fat or vice versa. At other times, they use complex chemicals as the substitute. Either way, your health and waistline suffers.

18. **Avoid your triggers.** Back when I smoked cigarettes, I always had one after every meal. Eating became a trigger for my smoking habit. Some places and things can be your overeating triggers. Perhaps it is just Saturday football games. If so, you need to plan in advance what you are going to do to curb those cravings while watching the game. Maybe you could have a couple of bowls of carrots and cauliflower handy.

19. **If your family has some favorite restaurants, make sure you have a meal plan even before someone suggests going there.** Study the menu for foods that are filling, but not completely dangerous to meeting and maintaining your weight goals.

20. **No fast food for the rest of your life.** If necessary, take a sack lunch to work.

21. **Create a "Snack Food List" of items to curb your cravings without busting your waist line.** Keep the list available in a noticeable place like the refrigerator

door. Then, make sure that you have virtually all those items available all the time, so you have a variety from which you may choose. BTW, it may be helpful for you to prepare your personal lists of healthy foods for breakfasts, lunches, and dinners. That will provide you with choices when your brain goes blank with food cravings.

22. **If the restaurant serves too much food per order, then have them put half of yours in a take out container for a later meal.** Depending on what the food is, it might be good to put it into a plastic bag and freeze it. That way, you can save time by microwaving it at another time.

23. **Brush your teeth immediately following your evening meal.** It will help you avoid after dinner snacks. If you need an evening snack, try something like sugar-free gelatin or a diet soft drink.

24. **Work toward being healthy, not just losing weight.** The result will be a lean, strong body and a happier life.

25. **Recruit family and friends to support the changes you need in order to keep the weight off.** Let's face it, in a family, your choices will affect them. Perhaps you can't resist a Snickers bar if it is in the house, it might be good if you never see one there. The kitchen, in particular, should be a "safe zone" where none of

your hot button foods ever go. Ever is a long time and may be a sacrifice for them since they aren't the one's struggling with keeping the weight down.

26. **Start increasing your level of activity to burn more calories each day.** Remember! If you burn 500 additional calories per day, that equals one pound per week of weight loss.

27. **Do NOT. I repeat, do NOT reward your weight loss success with your favorite foods.** Instead, buy yourself a piece of clothing you couldn't have worn before.

28. **Continue reading and studying about healthy eating and exercise practices.** Plan to read at least one internet article each week or one book per month about these subjects.

Appendix B
Basic Sources for Body Weight Exercises

These are by no means all the possible workouts that are suitable for weight loss, but they are a good beginning. As you click on these links, you should find plenty of related sites that can give you workout ideas.

A Beginner Body Weight Circuit to Burn Fat and Build Muscle
http://www.nerdfitness.com/blog/2009/12/09/beginner-body-weight-workout-burn-fat-build-muscle/

Beginner Body Weight Workouts
https://tribesports.com/workouts/beginner-bodyweight-routine

15 Best Body Weight Exercises for Men
http://www.mensfitness.com/training/build-muscle/15-best-bodyweight-exercises-men

50 Bodyweight Exercises You Can Do Anywhere
http://greatist.com/fitness/50-bodyweight-exercises-you-can-do-anywhere

25 Exercises You Need to Be Doing
http://www.popsugar.com/fitness/Body-Weight-Exercises-34376556

Also go to <u>YouTube.com</u> and search for "body weight exercises." You'll get videos that will teach you how to do some of the best ones with proper form. This site also has plenty of info about working out with gym equipment too. For rookies like me, it was a life-saver (if only I had started out with it instead of making some bad mistakes at the beginning).

Appendix C

Low Calorie Snacks to Prevent Food Cravings

How to Spot a Good Snack

There's no such thing as a perfect snack, but we want to know how to make some wise choices. Here are some suggestions:

Keep it to about 200 calories or less. That's enough to keep your metabolism working to burn up some of what you put in.

Look for lots of protein. High protein snacks help stimulate production of leptin, which will make you feel fuller. **Try to hit five grams of protein.** It's great if you can get five grams of protein in your snacks. I've even had times when I went to the frig and dug out a skinless, boneless chicken tenderloin that I had grilled for a previous meal. At 120 calories and 24 grams of protein, I was more than happy. I love grilled chicken!

Check out the fiber. Fiber is great as a snack because it is slow to digest. It also expands in your stomach when you drink water with it. Try to hit the 3 gram level of fiber in your snacks. My chicken tenderloin had exactly zero. Oh, well, nobody's perfect.

Watch the fat! Do not exceed 12 grams of fat in your snack. There went my Snickers® bar... well, not actually. I could have a Snickers® because it only has 9.9 grams of fat. But it is loaded down with 18.2 grams of sugar! Maybe I could settle for a granola bar with only 90 calories, 1.5 grams of fat, but oh, no just 1 gram of protein!

When choosing your snack, it's great to have a tool like MyFitnessPal because you can look at your nutritional balance for the day. If you are low on protein, emphasize protein in your snack. If you have too much fat, you might want a fat-free snack like an apple.

List of Snack Ideas (Have them on Hand)

1. Fruits like apples, bananas, pears, oranges, tangerines, grapes, or tomatoes.

2. Protein bars and shakes.

3. Nuts like almonds, peanuts, pistachios, cashews, chestnuts, soy nuts, and walnuts

4. Homemade egg salad sandwich (1 hard boiled egg, 1 tsp mayo, a pinch of celery salt, 1 slice whole wheat bread)

5. Air popped popcorn with butter flavored canola oil spray and popcorn salt.

6. One cup of Raisin Bran with skim milk

7. KIND® Peanut Butter and Strawberry Bar

8. Grapes plus a stick of low fat Mozzarella string cheese

9. Small bowl of lentil vegetable soup (1 cup)

10. Dried fruits and berries, like apples, cranberries, raisins, blueberries

11. Oatmeal with fruit

12. Frozen yogurt with fruit

13. Raw vegetables like carrots, cauliflower, or broccoli. Used cold yogurt as a dip.

14. Homemade pumpkin yogurt (just mix vanilla yogurt with a couple of tablespoons f canned pumpkin and a pinch of pumpkin spice). Can you say pumpkin pie!

15. Applesauce (perhaps with flavorings)

16. Vanilla yogurt with fresh peach slices. (Apricots, strawberries, etc.)

17. Triscuits and homemade dip (mix small curd cottage cheese with plenty of mild salsa).

18. Pita Pizza.   (Cover a pita with marinara sauce, cut up low fat cheese sticks, diced onions, and Italian seasoning.

19. Baked chicken nuggets. Hand dipped in milk and floured.

20. Ham Roll. Roll two 97% fat free ham slices around mozzarella cheese stick. Only totals 110 calories!

21. Frozen banana chunks. Just buy the banana, cut it up, put it in a ZipLoc® bag and freeze. One medium banana is just 105 calories!

22. Blend banana with strawberries or raspberries, add just a touch of yogurt and freeze in small cups.

23. Blend non-fat yogurt with diet lemon-lime soda, then freeze. It's a non-fat, low calorie sherbert!

No doubt you can find hundreds more online. I've collected or created these for my own use during the period of weight loss.

Appendix D
Online Calculators to Aid Weight Loss

Calculate your BMR (Basal Metabolic Rate)
http://www.myfitnesspal.com/tools/bmr-calculator

Walking Distance and Calories Burned Calculator
http://walking.about.com/library/cal/uccalc2.htm

Body Fat Calculator
http://www.fitbie.com/fit_tools/body_fat

BMI Calculator
http://www.nhlbi.nih.gov/health/educational/lose_wt/BMI/b
micalc.htm

Calorie Calculator and Weight Loss Goals
http://www.healthyweightforum.org/eng/calculators/calories
-required/

Ideal Weight Calculator
http://www.calculator.net/ideal-weight-
calculator.html?ctype=standard&cage=66&csex=m&cheigh
tfeet=6&cheightinch=3&cheightmeter=180&printit=0&x=81
&y=17
*This Calculator gives ideal weights under several
different formulas. Results are above calculator.*

Recipe Nutrition Calculator
http://www.myfitnesspal.com/recipe/calculator
Just enter the recipe name, servings, ingredients and
quantities into the blank to calculate the calories in your
favorite homemade recipes

Bibliography

Guise, S. (2013). *Mini Habits: Smaller Habits, Bigger Results.* Deep Existence.

Hellmich, N. (2013, September 24). Weight loss can help reduce knee pain from arthritis. *USAToday Online.*

Johnson, C. (2012, May 25). *10 Eating Habits of the Highly Successful and Fit.* Retrieved from http://www.womenshealthmag.com/weight-loss/healthy-eating-habits

Matthews, J. (2014). *Beat the Diet Trap: Discover the Truth about Weight Loss and Learn How to Change the Habits of a Lifetime.* Archangelink.

National Institutes of Health, National Heart, Lung, and Blood Indentification, Evaluation, and Treatment of Overweight and Obese Adults.

If you believe that this book was helpful, I encourage you to share with others by leaving a review on Amazon at http://www.amazon.com//dp/B00OH01XYQ/

If you are interested in gaining more of the same perspective on weight loss, please go to my blog at www.mgwebb.net and click the link for weight loss.

Other books by Gary Webb include:

Free Indeed: A Devotional for Saints Who Still Struggle with Sin

With This Ring: Marriage Through the Eyes of Its Creator

and

The Meaning of the Cross: Its Impact on Your Life